AF596113

Warriors
of
Weight
The quickest method to chisel abs

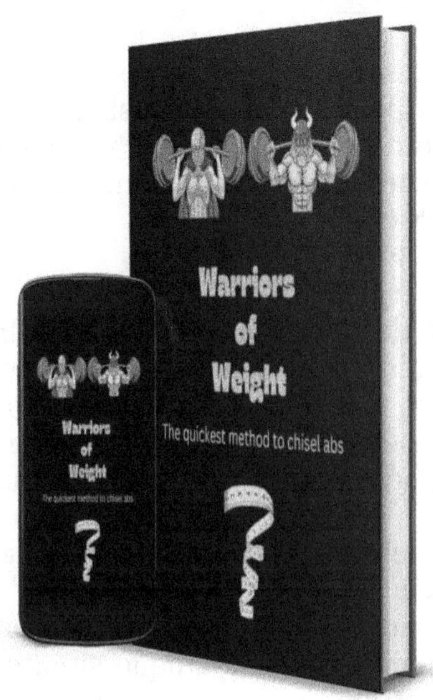

By AK Sawon

Terms and Conditions

LEGAL NOTICE

Despite making every effort to be as precise and thorough as possible, the Publisher does not at any time guarantee or suggest that the contents of this report are correct due to the Internet's tendency to change quickly.

Although every effort has been made to ensure the accuracy of the information in this publication, the publisher disclaims liability for any mistakes, omissions, or incorrect interpretations of the subject matter. Any perceived slights made towards particular individuals, organizations, or groups are unintended.

Like everything else in life, there are no guarantees of financial security in books offering practical guidance. Readers are advised to make decisions based on their own assessments of their unique situations and take appropriate action.

This book is not meant to be used as a source for accounting, financial, legal, or business advice. All readers are urged to consult with qualified experts in the disciplines of law, business, accounting, and finance.

This book is recommended for printing for ease of reading.

Table of Contents

Foreword

Let's be honest, buddy. Nothing about those turtlenecks is helping you get rid of that double chin. Next, have you ever experienced...

Sluggish? A bad shape? Do your clothes seem to be growing out of you more quickly than they ought to? Find all the details you require right here.

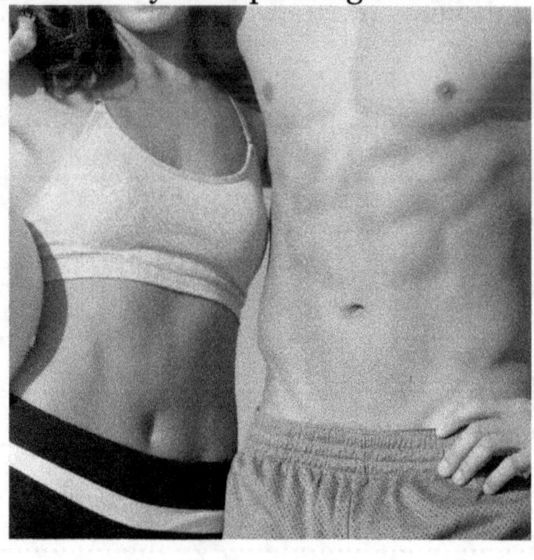

Warriors of Weight

By **AK Sawon**

Chapter 1:

Introduction

summary

Are you the kind of person who always has a bowl of crisps in front of him and a bottle of beer poised on his stomach while watching TV while daydreaming about a delicious, greasy Big Mac and hating yourself for it?

Are you sick and tired of being overweight? Do you desire to move in the appropriate direction and have these inquiries end? Well, you got it, buddy!

We'll get you up and running in no time with this copy of Weight Warriors: The Spartan's Guide to Chiseled Abs! since it is now that you should decide to lead a healthy lifestyle.

The Foundation

But above all, keep in mind that being healthy does not necessarily mean being in shape. The condition of being in good physical, mental, and spiritual health. Not how you choose to rank demons or how cute you look in your new body-con blouse.

Making the proper decisions will undoubtedly lead to fantastic outcomes throughout your lifetime. Giving your body the workout and positive energy flow it need is what it all about. About reinventing oneself. transforming you into a more positive, joyful, and healthy individual. The adage "health is riches" has always been true.

Wellness is health. You don't have to spend money to be happy.

If you have been overweight for the bulk of your life or if one of your parents is obese, genetics may play a substantial role in your obesity.

However, this is not a death sentence since, as I can guarantee you, hard work and lots of exercise will pay off. Right now, we can eliminate the fat gene and those fat cells.

Adopting the lovely idea of being physically fit can have many wonderful benefits, such as the wonderful sensation you'll have when you wake up one morning and feel completely refreshed,

improved over your previous state. It's like always getting out of bed on the right side. And when you notice the pounds dropping off the scale, it feels like Christmas arrived early. You'll be able to run that additional mile you thought you'd never be able to finish or fit back into your beloved jeans that you outgrew last year. And things improve.

Living a healthy lifestyle is not something you can pick up or put down as you please. It requires commitment and tenacity. You will be able to make simple decisions that will make you successful and happy in a couple of weeks, if not even days.

The process of toning is excellent and gives you the extra push and assurance that everyone should possess. Keep in mind that leading a healthy lifestyle is a result of the decisions you make every day.

There is no secret technique; all it takes is commitment to make wise decisions in your life. Never think about maintaining or being demanding on your health.

Instead, consider your health as a wise investment rather than a daunting task. Keep in mind that we are talking about you. Additionally, don't you merit the very finest that life has to offer? You'll succeed in this race if you maintain your composure and confidence.

List your objectives. Set goals for yourself at regular intervals, such as once every few weeks, once every few months, and so on. Be unafraid. Step by step, together, we're completing this.

Write down your goals, such as running 5 kilometres in the next six months. High expectations and lofty dreams are nothing to be terrified of. You are the only thing in the way. Do not anticipate being able to run 5 miles on your first outing. Don't panic; you're just beginning off and your body isn't used to the strenuous action at hand.

Take things slowly and try not to be too hard on yourself. If you continually telling yourself that you aren't capable of doing something, you will never succeed. Get out from under those jogging shoes.

Time-wasting is the enemy.

Let's start with a nutritional and exercise notebook, in which you should record everything you eat and how much exercise you get each day. Keeping track will enable you to determine your progress, estimate weight fluctuations, and other things.

Keep in mind that everything adds up, from that extra latte at the coffee shop to climbing the stairs at work. Use this helpful notebook to identify your negative behaviors and areas that need work.

It's crucial to keep to the truth despite all the cutting-edge fitness innovations, extraordinary diets, and bizarre misconceptions. Begin by doing the simple things first, such as learning how to read nutrition labels, estimating your daily caloric intake, and avoiding eating too many fatty foods. This will assist you in making excellent dietary decisions.

Discover the possibilities for workout clubs and activities in your region by getting out there. Excellent strategies to start your physical quest and get fit include walking, swimming, and yoga.

Get rid of outdated lures. You become what you consume. It's time to let rid of the unhealthy eating practices. But this romance comes to a pleasant conclusion. Living a healthy lifestyle involves breaking harmful habits. Instead of starting from scratch with everything you do, take small, doable steps and achieve some early successes.

Be kind with yourself. You'll err occasionally. You're going to snap and consider ruining the whole situation by running to the nearest fast food restaurant and stuffing yourself savagely.

That's alright. All forms of rewards are beneficial, and occasional small treats are acceptable. Give yourself a break and only treat yourself when you feel you deserve it.

like a handful of Kisses the size of your palm that will genuinely satiate you after your evening run. However, if you're consistently cheating, you need to evaluate what's happening and figure out how to get back on track.

Keep in mind that the scale doesn't tell the complete story. Your personality, as well as how attractive, unattractive, or kind you are, are not determined by your weight.

The scale is there to make it easier for you to recognize the modifications you still need to make as well as the ones you've already made. Even while losing weight might be at the top of your priority list, other factors like eating more nutritiously every day and becoming happier and fitter are also crucial.

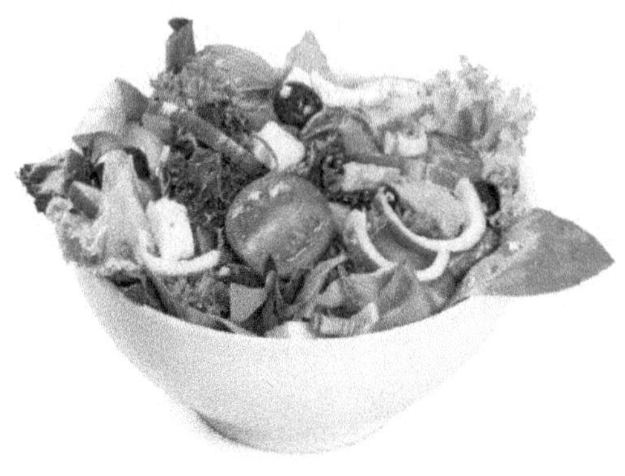

Chapter 2:

Getting Abs Through Food

summary

Is joining the celebrity diet everyone has been talking about your first choice when it comes to attaining those spectacular, A-list abs? Where do they get their strange jungle juice?

Sometimes you'll lose five to ten pounds quickly, but due of the sudden changes in your eating habits, your old eating habits will soon return.

You must make sure to be really committed to your diet if you're actually bent on losing those pounds. Don't stray from what you find comfortable. A diet is a way of life, not a special event.

The Meals

You won't be able to eat as many of the items you used to when you're on a diet. You have to be prepared to make a sacrifice, but it will all be worthwhile in the end. But fear not, for the lovely world of replacements and alternatives is here to assist.

Diets may compel you to eat things you don't enjoy, find comforting, or are difficult to digest.

But because of this, you must follow a diet that satisfies your nutritional requirements.

To avoid giving up after a few days, you'll need to be content and at ease with it. You must also like the meals because all of the vigorous exertion will work up an appetite.

Diet alone makes you want to scream loud enough for a horror movie. This is due to the misconception that diets involve bland food and deprivation, which is untrue. A diet is really just a better-portioned, healthier plate.

Therefore, it's time to quit settling for celery sticks at gatherings while everyone else is having a blast filling their faces with those crab puffs.

Given how important food is to how we interact with one another, it is time to stop avoiding social situations. when you see food that you would love to consume
but are unable to do so due to the fear of having to deal with it while the others don't have to worry about a thing. As a result, we feel depleted, alone, and insecure. Now that we're attempting to get better, it's time to quit feeling so horrible. a totally different, happier, and healthier person.

Studies have found risks in the yo-yo dieting cycle of weight loss. losing, gaining again, losing and gaining it back plus a little more. Wide variations in body weight are taxing to the body. Every time, we worry that we won't get it back, but statistics prove that the majority of us will. And the concept is risky and wild as a whole.

The diet initially provides you a sense of control. Your eating habits are under your control. Success may be seen as the scale declines. But soon you're up against hunger pangs, cravings for forbidden foods, and a lack of energy brought on by the reduced calorie intake. You eventually rebel against the diet and start "cheating." And before you know it, you're back to your old habits and midnight nibbles.

We would all prefer to avoid relapsing.

When you consume less calories, your body slows down your metabolism. It's essential to burn less calories each day if you want to keep your body's processes going.

It is advisable to continue with a slow, steady system. Don't rush things because even the smallest adjustments can cause your body to respond. Being kind to our body is
paramount importance Lean muscle mass will be lost along with fat and water weight if activity is not added to the diet. Your metabolism slows down even more as a result of muscle loss, so you'd need to consume even fewer calories each day to keep losing weight.

Maintaining an exercise routine while on a diet requires conscious effort. Without exercise, you'll stray from your diet and, worse yet, gain weight more quickly because your body will burn less calories each day. Even worse, rather than the muscle you lost, the weight will return as fat. Your body will appear even less toned and wholesome than before.

For this reason, every diet must have a positive dynamic with exercise.

As a first step to improving your health and looks, start exercising every day.

It's not necessary to undertake rigorous exercise. Choose activities you enjoy doing, such as riding, swimming, or walking. gives your body a good workout most days of the week, leaving one day for you to recover from all the toning your body is doing.

Look for a 100-calorie change you can do this week. Maybe it's consuming one fewer can of soda each day or substituting fat-free milk for cream in your coffee.

Instead of that unhealthy bag of chips, reach for a baked potato, or pass on the buttercream cupcake in favor of a modest plate of apple and cheese. You can significantly improve your eating habits if you make a 100-calorie modification each week for the next six weeks.

Don't think of it as depriving yourself of the foods you enjoy; instead, consider it as cutting out calories that you could live without much better. You can shift your energy balance to favor lean muscle growth and maintenance while simultaneously burning and losing fat by making these changes. Don't you just love the sound of that now?

Instead of being abrupt, this will be progressive. After a while, you'll start to realize that your clothes are fitting more comfortably, your waist is getting smaller, and you have more energy. The new suite you've been itching to go into is now available for purchase.

The difference will be obvious to friends who haven't seen you in a long. The best part is that you didn't endure a torturous diet; instead, you properly nourished your body with healthier food alternatives and vigorous activity. You rock, champ!

Chapter 3:

It's More Important to Understand Why Than How

summary

It's time to think of some enjoyable activities to do instead of that incredibly cheesy, party-sized pizza. Since it's a little challenging, let's start with a simpler request.

It's usually a good idea to include some form of accompanying physical activity when deciding what to eat for breakfast, lunch, or dinner.

For instance, you could have a leisurely stroll across the park after supper. To cultivate the best mindset for weight loss, it is essential to drill the idea of exercising after meals.

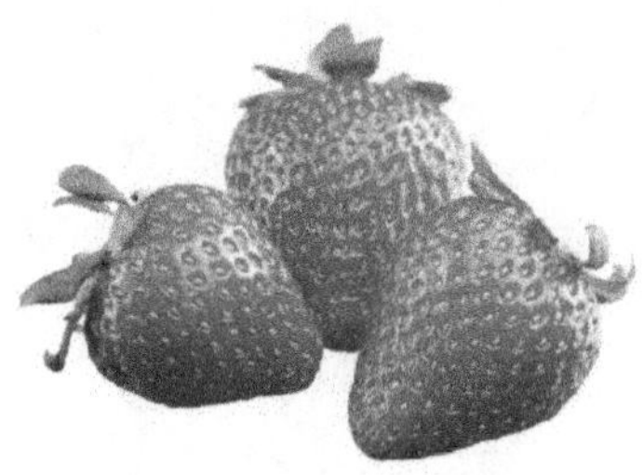

Look here

Change Your Thought Processes

Exercise from home may be far more convenient than stepping outside of your comfort zone and striving to make time to get to the gym because physical activity works best when it's a consistent part of your life.

What could be better than performing all the demanding activities in the security and comfort of your own home? Additionally, physical exercise is frequently more enjoyable when it occurs in a comfortable setting. Exactly.

You will be more likely to persist with simple exercise routines and advance to more strenuous physical activity more quickly if you start out with them.

Many of us are addicted to our cars, but if we just make a small adjustment and choose to walk instead of take a ride, we might be able to transform running errands into an excellent workout. Why not walk or ride a bicycle to the nearby grocery store instead of driving?

Try substituting casual jogging and quick walks for your usual drive-through throughout town. By doing this, you will not only be able to significantly reduce your gas costs, but you will also be assisting Mother Nature rather than adding to pollution. Amazing, I know.

Instead of using the elevator in your apartment building, use the steps. jog the dog of your neighbor. Enter a fun run. There are so many enjoyable methods to exercise!

Great if you have any children! Children like to play and move about. Get your kids to join you while you walk instead of loading up the minivan with the entire family. Excellent workout and clean air are amazing.

Another great approach to squeeze in as much exercise as you can is to multitask.

Get a wireless handheld so you can talk to your pal as you lift weights. This is covert and powerful.

Vacuuming and dusting jobs that require standing up don't have to be unpleasant anymore. Consider performing them a few times each day. If you can, use ankle weights and take brief "walking breaks" to extend your legs.

Every time you enter or leave a room, perform five or ten pushups. Just a few seconds to get your motor going, nothing more.

When it comes to physical activity, a lot of people see their television as the enemy, but that doesn't have to be the case. Consider how much time you spend watching television on the couch, and then imagine putting yourself on a treadmill while you watch. Presto!

Make one of your favorite shows your "physical activity show," which you watch while exercising. The optimal length for a fantastic workout is an hour-long program, which lasts 45 minutes without commercials. Many shows are available for purchase or rental on DVD.

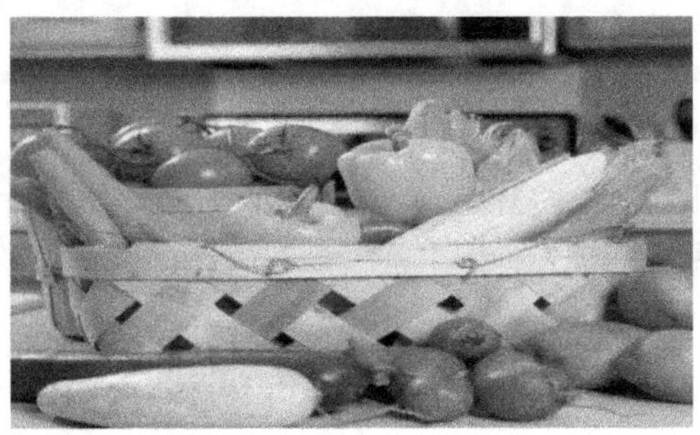

Chapter 4:

Beginner-Friendly

Exercises

summary

You want the best fitness plans to help you enhance your entire physical appearance when you're searching for them.

A fitness regimen that improves your overall health is what you seek. On the other hand, no fitness routine intended to help you lose weight is simple or painless.

The efficiency of your workout program will not at all work for shape, toning, or weight loss if the exercises you perform do not cause you any pain. It is the person executing it, not the software, who is at fault when something goes wrong.

No gain without pain.

Get to it!

To achieve your goals in any workout regimen, you must understand what is required of you:

1) You must be sufficiently and effectively motivated by the program to reduce the number of calories you consume and increase the number of calories you burn each day.

2) The regimen should be followed slowly and steadily to lose weight. For the first several weeks, you must reasonably drop 1 pound per week.

3) If you have never exercised before, start out slowly and gradually increase the duration and intensity of your workouts as your body adjusts.

4) While exercising, it's crucial to have fun while doing it. Pick workouts that you like and that fit your personality as a whole.

5) To get the maximum health benefits and weight loss, the exercise program should be followed regularly; ideally, make it a daily practice. Pick the pursuits that work with your schedule.

6) Workout with comfort. Comfort is important. If you're at ease, you're having fun. If you enjoy the exercise, you'll workout for longer periods of time, burning off more fat.

7) Your comfort and safety should always come first when exercising. Meaning that you must dress and wear shoes that are a perfect fit for you in order to work well without disruption or distraction.

8) There are many different workouts you may pick from, so switch things up every day to avoid getting bored.

9) Make an effort. It's crucial to raise your intensity and length during each exercise. The impact increases as you perform it more frequently. Additionally, treat yourself to whatever you want once you've accomplished your goals. Never give up on yourself or your ability to reduce weight, and take pleasure in your workouts. Include that exercise in your daily routine. Keep in mind that weight loss is possible and will happen if you only believe in it and exercise.

Here are some exercise plans for losing weight for you.

Perform the fundamental warm-up exercises prior to beginning the activity to avoid cramps, strained muscles, and pain. Exercises to cool down afterward are similar.

Broad Squat

Spread your legs out wide as you stand upright. Make certain you can distribute it evenly.

Raise your arms in the shape of a Y above your head.

By pushing your hips back, slowly squat down; maintain this position for as long as you can; then return to the starting position.

Perform as many wide squats as you can, up to 15.

You might be able to hold a squat for longer as you get stronger.

Do pushups

Lie on the ground with your face downward.

Grasp your shoulders with your hands.

Pushing against the floor, slowly lift your body off the ground with the aid of your hands and feet. Keep your body upright while performing this.

To lessen the strain on the arms for novices, rise your body from your knees as opposed to your feet.

Make it 5 counts for 3 sets if you are unable to complete 15 repeats.

Leaps and Jumps

Stand up straight with your arms at your sides.

Spread your legs wide as you jump, raising your arms

above your head in a circular motion as your hands come together above.

Put your arms back at your sides and stand up once more. Make around 60 repetitions.

Chapter 5:
Raising the Bar With Your Workouts

summary

This chapter intensifies your workouts.

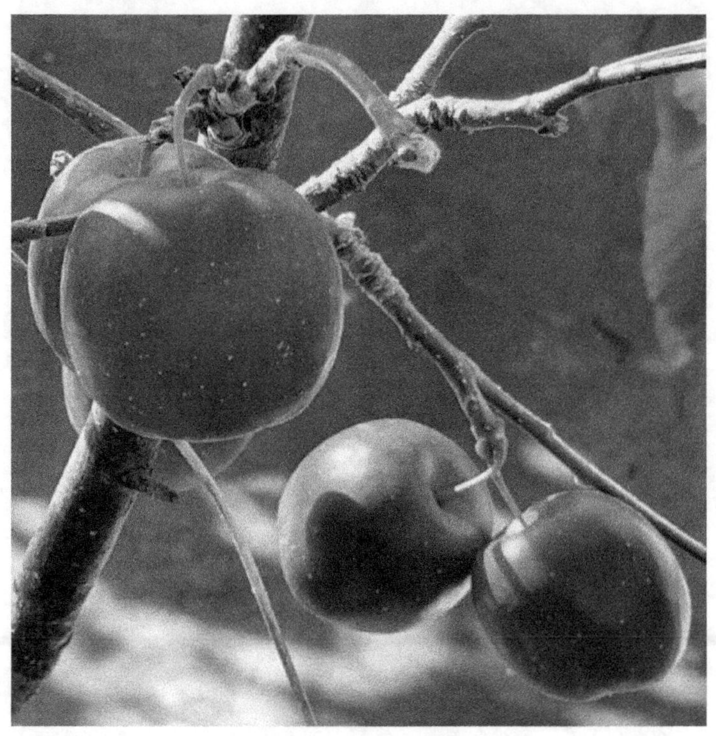

It Altering

INTERMEDIATE

False Fly

- Pick up two dumbbells. You decide the weight, but don't go too light or heavy.
- Lie on the ground with your head raised.
- Raise the dumbbells slowly until they are over your chest. Keep your arms straight at all times.
- Next, slowly descend to the ground while maintaining a slight elevation off of it.
- 15 times or as long as you can withstand it should be repeated.

Shoulder Press

- The only difference between this position and lying flat is that you are holding the dumbbells at ear level.

Seated Triceps Extension

- Straighten your back and lift a dumbbell with both hands above your head.

- Verify that the weight is neither excessively light or heavy.
- Still holding the dumbbell in both hands behind your back, lower it gradually.

- Attempt to keep the raised arms vertical.
- Return to the beginning posture and carry out 15 sitting triceps extensions there.

One Armed Row

- Lean forward while supporting your body with your left arm on a chair with your left knee placed there. Your right hand should be holding a dumbbell. By extending your arm toward the ceiling, lift the weight. Hold. Return to the beginning. Perform 15 repetitions.

Dumbbell Bicep Curl

- takes one of two positions: standing or sitting.
- Each hand should be holding a dumbbell as you lower it to the ground.
- Lift the right dumbbell slowly in the direction of your chest.
- As you raise the dumbbell, curl it so that your palm is facing your chest.
- On the opposite side, repeat the action. 15 bicep curls with a dumbbell.

ADVANCED

Walking lunge while twisting the torso

- Standing is a good place to start.
- Step forward and bring your hips down.
- Twist your upper body in the direction of the side of the stretched leg once you are fully positioned. Return to your starting position by turning around to the front.
- Follow the same procedure on the opposite side.

High Plank

- Start out by doing a push-up with your hands shoulder-width apart from your shoulders.
- Maintain the straightest back you can.
- Maintain for 15 seconds.
- Side Lunge with Arms Raised
  Pose yourself upright.
- Straighten your arms in front of you.
- Step with your right foot to the side, then

slowly lower your hips.

- Go back to the starting point.
- Perform 5 times, and then switch to the other leg.

Chapter 6:

Secret Techniques for Burning Fat

summary

While some people starve themselves, others exercise frequently. While some people watch the hands on the clock move while pounding the pavement in the gym, others choose the expensive shortcut of surgical interventions.

If you want to lose weight and keep it off, which is inhumanly impossible, it takes a lot of effort. Our lives revolve around enjoying delicious food and feeling good about ourselves. As a result, we work out to maintain the type of figure we desire.

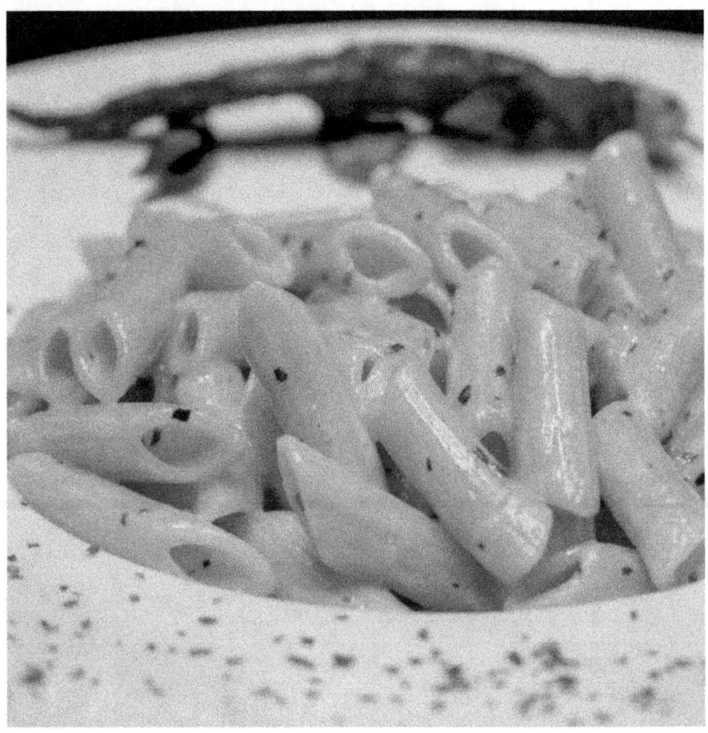

Excellent Information

Just because something is challenging at first doesn't imply you won't eventually be able to enjoy it. There is a big difference between working hard because you feel obligated to and working hard because it's something you really want.

As discussed throughout the entire book, choosing to live a healthy lifestyle. If you are motivated enough, you are entitled to and deserve it. Losing those pounds won't seem as difficult with the help of these top-secret fat-burning tricks. And when you put all of your effort into improving your health, the results are beautiful.

Watch out for: 1) Timely Eating Eating! Everybody's preferred pastime. If you have some self-control, doing this is the easiest thing to do. Your body breaks down food as you eat it, and depending on what you eat, it may or may not eventually stop burning fat. You're doing OK if you consume a balanced diet that includes meals high in protein and natural carbohydrates. However, dietary habits are as crucial.

Instead of simply two or three large meals, make sure to eat smaller, more frequent meals that are balanced throughout the day. Your metabolism will continue to run throughout the day if you eat little and often. You can prevent overeating by eating little snacks throughout the day.

Suppertime, as it is best to avoid eating after 6 o'clock in the evening. To prevent unexpected binges in the middle of the night or during the day, observe correct meal times as well. After lunch, a salad can quickly fill you up.

2) Develop a Plan

Everyone wants to look their best and lose a few pounds. What's the aim? Five pounds to go? Whatever your objective, it's critical to decide on it early on and then create a strategy for achieving it. This need not be complicated. Saying that you wish to shed one pound per week for fifteen weeks can be sufficient. You may maintain your focus and clarity during your weight loss time by keeping this straightforward goal in mind each day of the week. Keep moving forward if you can see the finish line! Move forth, soldier!

3) Breakfast

It's true what they say: "The most essential meal of the day is breakfast." Since you are not eating while you are asleep, your metabolism is greatly slowed. Your metabolism needs to be reset when your day begins so that you can start burning fat straight away.

Otherwise, your body would continue to drag on as if it were still in a state of slumber, preventing you from losing the weight you need to. Every morning, eat a healthy breakfast that is high in protein and carbohydrates to help your body get going. The ideal way to start the day is with a breakfast fit for a king. And progressively consume less food during the day. According to another proverb, "For Eat your breakfast like a king. Eat like a knight for lunch. Eat like a slave for dinner as well."

4) Resistance

Healthy eating is important, but it won't be enough on its own. You must exercise, and resistance training is one of the most crucial components of fitness. You should do this three times a week, with a day of recovery in between each workout, so get to the gym or grab some weights for a solid workout at home. You'll soon notice a significant difference in your energy level and the amount of weight you're losing if you work your way up to 60 minute sessions.

Some of the most frequent questions on Earth already know the solutions, while some of the bigger problems in life may never have an answer. These tried-and-true fat-burning suggestions. They have been tested, and you can trust them. Just consider your objectives and consider how these fat-burning suggestions will help you get there. The goalposts are almost in sight.

A Conclusion

This method of living necessitates wise decisions. You'll find remarkable outcomes if you're willing to persevere. I guarantee that this independence brings unbounded joy that pressures in the outside world are unable to.

Your inherent sense of goodness is delight. It is a sacred birthright for you. Everyone ought to be content. What better way to start than by beginning to make these excellent life decisions? We all deserve to be.

When you begin to identify with who you are and link your life to greater goals in the pursuit of improving yourself, amazing things begin to happen. There will be a ton of support available.

You can always count on the universe to support you and provide for your needs. People and opportunities will start to appear everywhere. As you start to distance yourself from your toxic connections and totally devote yourself to good health, coincidences and miracles start to happen.

Once you experience sensations of tranquility, harmony, and contentment, you will know you have arrived. You won't have issues with eating or weight anymore.

You'll be joyfully participating in life's dance. You'll know you've found yourself when you're fiercely alive with the glow of supreme contentment.

The wonder that has always been inside of you will finally start to shine through, and you'll be overcome with it.

And right now, it very certainly can. Because you're much fitter, healthier, and more self-assured now.

You are a unique individual, and you merit better. You're welcome, stormtrooper! You've reached the finishing line!

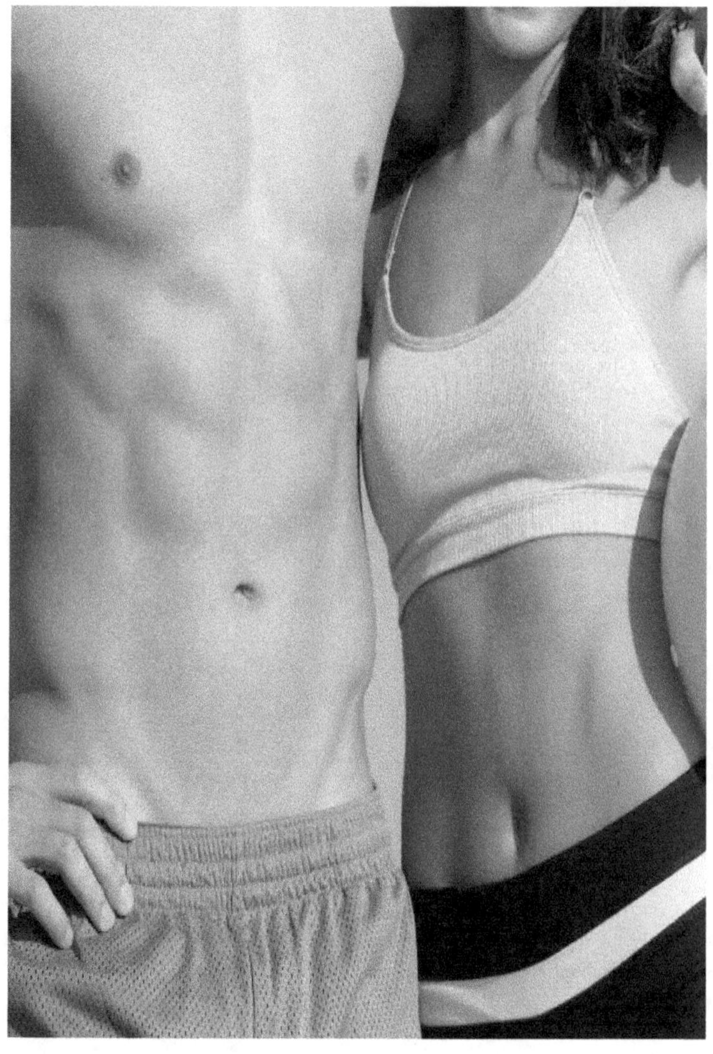

www.ingramcontent.com/pod-product-compliance
Lightning Source LLC
LaVergne TN
LVHW012034160826
845678LV00013B/2587

* 9 7 9 8 3 6 7 8 0 2 2 9 0 *